Medical Appraisal, Selection and Revalidation—
A Professional's Guide to Good Practice

To Susie and Anne

Medical Appraisal, Selection and Revalidation — A Professional's Guide to Good Practice

John Gatrell
BA (Hons) PGCE FCIPD MIMgt
Deputy Head
Bournemouth University Business School,

Tony White
PhD FRCS AKC
Consultant Otolaryngologist
Visiting Professor Bournemouth University

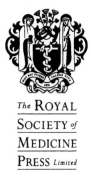

The ROYAL
SOCIETY of
MEDICINE
PRESS Limited

© 2001 Royal Society of Medicine Press Ltd
Reprinted 2001
1 Wimpole Street, London W1G 0AE, UK
207 Westminster Road, Lake Forest, IL 60045, USA
www.rsmpress.co.uk

British Library Cataloguing in Publication Data
A catalogue record for this book is available from the British Library

ISBN: 1-85315-400-8

Phototypeset by Phoenix Photosetting, Chatham, Kent

Printed in Great Britain by Bell and Bain Ltd, Glasgow

▶ Contents

5. SELECTION   33

▶ Preface

Since 1992 we have conducted a range of projects which were aimed at improving understanding of the non-clinical work of doctors. A large-scale survey of doctors was published by the National Health Service Training Directorate (NHSTD) in 1995 as *Medical Student to Medical Director—A Development Strategy for Doctors.* In preparation for this text we have drawn on documentation from the National Health Service Executive, the Medical Royal Colleges, British Medical Association (BMA), Standing Committee on Postgraduate Medical Education (SCOPME), British Association of Medical Managers (BAMM), Deaneries, Trusts and other related organisations from around the country. Our research has included observation of more than six hundred medical interviews and many meetings with panel members and chairs to discuss their approach. This work has led to the development and delivery of over three hundred training workshops on the practice of interviewing for appraisal and selection. These workshops have enabled us to collect and disseminate examples of good practice from a wide range of organisations around the country. This book assembles in one document a guide to good practice in the use of interviews in appraisal and selection. Most of the principles and core skills apply equally to many other one-to-one situations, such as taking histories and coaching. All the examples used in this book are taken from real interviews.

► Acknowledgements

We are grateful for the help, advice and support of the following:

Dr Clair du Boulay, Director of Medical Education, Southampton University Hospitals Trust;
Dr Shelley Heard, Postgraduate Dean, North Thames Deanery;
Dr Hugh Platt, Secretary, Royal College of Pathologists;
Dr Frank Smith, Associate Dean, General Practice, Wessex Deanery;
Dr Richard Weaver, Talbot Medical Centre
Professor Graham Winyard, Dean, PGMDE Wessex Deanery;
Dr Jenny Eaton, Associate Dean, South West Deanery;
Pam Corsie, Bournemouth University Business School, who, among many other contributions, ensured the workshops happened;
over 2000 consultants who attended our workshops and shared their experience and opinions with us, together with non-exective directors, lay chairs and postgraduate deans; and
numerous senior house officers who volunteered to help us by role-playing themselves in mock interviews.

►1
Introduction

Our normal, everyday working lives contain countless face-to-face meetings with individuals and small groups. We seldom ask ourselves if we are conducting an 'interview', but see ourselves as simply eliciting, or passing on, information. Many of these interactions can, however, have an important influence on work achievements. They may be aimed at getting information about a patient, or a future colleague, or to assess, or appraise, the performance of a trainee doctor, or even a colleague. In almost every case, the successful conclusion of interviews is almost entirely dependent on the skill with which they are undertaken. An interview is a conversation with a purpose. Although we speak of 'formal' interviews, the most effective are, in almost every case, conducted with a degree of informality. They should feel more than anything like normal conversation to the participants—interviewers and interviewees alike.

We review issues for a number of situations that commonly arise in the professional career of doctors—as trainee or trainer, junior or senior, as clinician or clinical manager. Our experience is based on research into the conduct of interviews in a range of settings. We have also been involved in conducting, and training others in a range of interview situations, including selection, appraisal, one-to-one teaching, disciplinary hearings and career counselling.

Communications skills are too often grouped under one heading. However, they are more usefully broken down into a number of different sets of skills. For example, classroom teaching requires a quite different approach from breaking bad news. Each is concerned with effective communication. Much of face-to-face communication is in the way we behave, as well as in our choice of words. Dealing with frightened or angry patients or relatives demands behaviours which would be out of place in a selection interview. We have tried to provide insight into the kinds of behaviours, language and approaches which are relevant to a wide range of interviews.

Communication can be shown as a process affected by a number of elements. It is often shown, as in Figure 1.1, as a set of stages which help, and hinder, the process.

In its simplest form, the start of a communication is an idea in the mind of the sender, which is to be aimed at the mind of a receiver. The idea must first be encoded. This usually means that the sender must find words which adequately describe the idea. In an interview setting, the sender then speaks the words. Noise describes any disturbance which might distort the message. This could be an external interruption to the interview, thoughts passing across the mind of the receiver, such as worries about what was said previously, or sounds which distract, or affect the receiver's hearing.

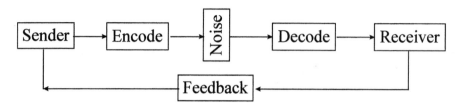

Figure 1.1 The communication process.

The receiver decodes the words, giving them his or her own interpretation. If there are differences in level of intelligence, learning or culture between the interviewee and interviewer, then interpretation can cause major problems. It may be a patient's inability to find words which describe a symptom, or a trainee whose nervousness in the presence of an examiner makes interpretation difficult.

It has been suggested that only 20–30% of the message we receive, or send, in a face-to-face communication is in the words we use. The rest is in non-verbal cues, such as the tone of voice, facial expression, body posture and level of eye contact. These non-verbal indicators may be represented as the 'noise' in Figure 1.1. They can radically affect the message received, often without our realising it.

The medical profession ensures that those entering it are properly scrutinised for suitability by proper and effective use of selection techniques. Revalidation has been introduced, among other objects, to promote good medical practice. Appraisal is an element within that process, the purpose of which is to 'support doctors in maintaining and improving their professional performance' (GMC, 2000). The appraisal meeting normally takes place annually, and is only as effective as the skills of those undertaking it. This book focuses on the development of capability in these critical areas of activity in medicine.

▶2
Core interviewing skills

This book seeks to provide you with grounding in the core aspects of inter-viewing. It does this by taking you through the supporting skills and the struc-ture of appraisal and selection interview settings. The core skills are relevant to a wider range of interview situations, for example history taking and research interviews as well. These are shown in Figure 2.1.

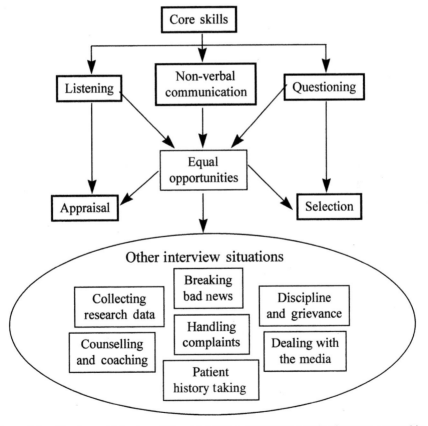

Figure 2.1 Structure of interview skills and settings showing the main elements covered in this book.

As interviewer, you will normally provide the meeting with its direction and tone. You achieve your purpose by asking questions, listening and giving information. Your behaviour, as well as your choice of words, are part of the process. These make up the core skills of interviewing, which are explored below.

Questioning

The interviewer has a limited range of 'tools' with which to guide and direct the interviewee towards the goals of the interview. The single most important of these is the use of questions. A clear understanding of the use of different types of question is a prerequisite to success. It should be noted, however, that getting the words right is a relatively small part of the process. The manner, tone of voice, facial expression and posture all go together with the words to affect the interviewee's willingness to 'open up' when being questioned. This is discussed in more detail below.

Types of questions and their uses

Experiential or situational questions

In most cases, the interviewer is seeking to understand the interviewee better. In our research into interviews, we have observed that questions which focus on the interviewee's past experience tend to be the most revealing. This requires skill in framing questions which 'draw out' the interviewee. The answers are then probed in order to gain deeper insight into the person's past behaviour patterns, motives, values, attitudes and personality. Thus, an approach that uses *open* questions, followed by *probing* and *reflective* questions, is likely to be most successful. This approach is explained in detail below.

The candidate must be given time to think of the example, even though this usually results in a quiet moment, or silence in the interview.

Open questions

Open-ended questions generate discussion and allow interviewers the opportunity to probe for facts and clarifications of details. They are used for exploring, gathering information and encouraging the candidate to talk freely. Open questions oblige the interviewee to respond with a full answer—they do not permit a 'Yes' or 'No' response. They are likely to start with 'Why. . .' or 'How. . .' or 'Tell me about. . .'.

Where opinions are being sought, or greater insight into the interviewee's situation or motives is needed, then it often helps to start a line of questioning by getting the interviewee to talk to you in their own words. Examples of open questions are:

'Tell me about your present job.'

'How would you describe the pain?'

'How can I help you?'

'Why did you choose to undertake research?'

Closed questions

These are useful when checking facts. They are phrased so that they usually elicit a 'Yes' or 'No' response. You may need to use closed questions to be absolutely sure that you have the information you need, or to confirm that you have understood a previous response.

'Was the paper published?'

'Did you pass the examination?'

'Have you carried out a tracheotomy by yourself?'

'Do you have a cough?'

A series of such questions results in the interviewer doing most of the talking, with the candidate answering briefly or only with 'Yes' or 'No'. Inexperienced interviewers can get trapped into a series of these questions, as they do not allow sufficient time for the interviewer to frame the next question properly. In history taking, closed questions may lead patients to give answers which match the doctor's assumptions, rather than the patient's real symptoms.

Probing questions

The open question elicits a full answer which provides the material for further exploration. Our observations of medical interviews suggested that, while many doctors knew how to employ open questions, the answers they elicited were seldom followed up, or probed. Use probing questions to explore in greater detail actions, events, experiences and associated feelings which have been mentioned by the candidate in their answers:

Open question: 'Think of an example where you successfully influenced your colleagues and changed their practice?';

Probing questions: . . . 'What happened then?' . . . 'How did you react?' . . . 'What did he/she say?' . . . 'Why do you think that approach worked?'

Open question: 'Think of an occasion when you had to communicate unpleasant news to someone';

Probing questions: . . . 'What was the end result?' . . . 'How did you achieve it?' . . . 'How did you feel?' . . . 'What did you do then?'

Open question: 'Tell me about a time when you had to do something you felt unsure about?';

Probing questions: . . . 'How did you go about it?' . . . 'What was the result?' . . . 'What did you learn from that?' . . . 'How would you approach it next time?'

Open question: 'Tell me about your illness';

Probing questions: . . . 'When did it start?' . . . 'Where did it hurt most?' . . . 'Describe the pain.' . . . 'How long did it last?'

Interrupting

A confident interviewee will take over a subject and may even keep talking in order to avoid further questions. This happens, typically, in the following way.

Open question: 'Tell me about your research.'

In a selection interview, the answer may take up the full time allowance of that panel member while the candidate describes the background, aims and content of the research. The technical nature of the answer rarely adds to the panel's understanding of the candidate. We have observed that the questioner seldom interrupts to avoid this time wasting.

Other panel members quickly demonstrate boredom as the candidate develops the answer. This quickly has a negative effect on the whole interview.

Our recommendation is that candidates are unaffected by interruptions, as long as they demonstrate continuing interest in the candidate.

Thus, a further, probing question—'What do you feel you gained from the work?'—inserted at a time when the candidate has drawn a breath, will bring out information about the candidate rather than their research. This may be

followed, for example, by 'How would you do it differently
next time?'

Interruptions are usually acceptable if they are in the form of a probing question, and the interviewer continues to show interest in the interviewee. This approach requires careful listening, and some practice, if it is to work well.

Reflective questions

These enable the interviewer to check understanding and to elicit further information about a particular aspect of an interviewee's most recent response, perhaps about sensitive aspects of their experience. They involve selecting a word, or a few words, from the interviewee's most recent response, and feeding them back as a question. They encourage the interviewee to continue talking, without asking directly:

'You felt unsure?'

'You were worried?'

'You felt *severe* pain?'

'You took responsibility for the patient?'

These questions work well in counselling situations, but can also be powerful in getting interviewees in selection or appraisal interviews to go into greater depth regarding their motives and feelings.

At the end of a response to an open question it can be effective to wait for a few seconds to allow the interviewee to continue to give more detail, or to expand on the last point made.

A small gesture may be used, or you may merely add a comment such as

'And...?'

'So...?'

'Go on...'

'Tell me more'.

Leading questions

These are seldom, if ever, helpful to the interviewer. Interviewers sometimes seek to help the candidate to understand by first setting their question in context. For example, they might say:

'Hello. I shall be concentrating on your team-working
strengths. How well do you fit into teams?'

> 'Patients with this complaint frequently say they get pains in the stomach. Do you ever suffer from stomach-ache?'

These are questions that suggest a particular answer—one which the interviewer may expect to hear. This is unhelpful in all but a very limited set of circumstances, and should be avoided, particularly when taking a patient's history, or in selection interviews. It is better to keep the question open, with no hint as to the expected response. This ensures the information gained is more useful to the interviewer.

Multiple questions

Another trap into which inexperienced interviewers frequently fall is triggered by their desire to be helpful to the interviewee. They worry that their first attempt at wording a question may be misunderstood by the interviewee, so they re-state the question in a different way. In elaborating their first attempt, they end up asking a second question. This invariably causes confusion.

> 'What was the subject of your project?' . . . 'Was it a difficult choice?' . . . 'How did you make the decision in the end?' . . . 'Did you have any help with the decision?'

> 'When you were in this situation with your colleague who had a problem, did you confront her directly?' . . . 'or was it on an informal basis after the meeting?' . . . 'what did she say?' . . . 'did it resolve the situation?'

or, when addressing a patient:

> 'How many times do you get up in the night to pass water?' . . . 'How good is the stream?' . . . 'How difficult is it to start the flow?' . . . 'Do you still feel you need to go afterwards?'

The subject is uncertain which question to answer first. Frequently, the series of questions ends with a closed question, as the examples above demonstrate. Ask one question at a time, and only clarify your question if the interviewee asks for help.

Non-verbal communication

Effective listening

People respond more effectively to interviewers who can be seen to be listening. Regular eye contact should be maintained throughout an interview, and occasional nods or sounds of approval are used to encourage the interviewee to continue developing full answers to the questions.

Listen with genuine interest, actively encourage the other person to talk and show understanding and empathy. This is the simplest skill to describe, yet the most difficult of skills to acquire. Good listening is more than just registering words like a tape recorder. If it were easy, more people would be good at it. The more you listen and the better you listen, the more confident interviewees feel about talking to you and the better your chances of helping them talk freely and openly to you.

Look at the interviewee as they are talking, and if they can see from the expression on your face that you are paying attention to everything they say, they will be encouraged to give full replies to your questions. If, on the other hand, you look away, or if they see boredom, lack of interest or disapproval in your expression, they will be much less inclined to speak openly and freely to you. Impatient interviewers may glance at their watch in an unguarded moment. This usually has a devastating effect on the interviewee's confidence and willingness to open up.

Using silence

We often feel uncomfortable if a long silence occurs during a conversation. This leads us to fill it, sometimes with a thoughtless contribution which does not add, and may detract, from an interview. Trainee doctors can find silence unsettling during a meeting with a patient, and therefore feel duty bound to say something. It is usually preferable to allow the patient to speak, and they will also feel the need to fill the silence.

Silence often has a positive effect in an interview. It can be used to put gentle pressure on an interviewee, and can be an effective way of getting at details which he or she may not otherwise have released. In selection interviews, this requires a discipline and common understanding not always found in inexperienced panel members, who must stop themselves from talking while the seconds pass.

Non-verbal behaviour in the interview

We make the assumption that on all but a very small number of occasions, you will wish to get interviewees to talk openly and freely about themselves or the situation they are describing. It has already been suggested that non-verbal cues form an important part of the communication between people in face-to-face situations. They can affect the interviewee by either encouraging, or discouraging, them from responding freely.

Positive listening involves looking at the person, nodding occasionally, smiling, and generally expressing approval of, and interest in, what they are saying. If you find that your interviewee will not stop talking, this may be because you are maintaining eye contact and nodding benignly. This transmits the message that you wish them to continue talking. A probing question can be used to redirect the interviewee.

Negative behaviours, such as checking your watch, reading notes (such as an application form), asides to fellow panel members or gazing out of a window while the interviewee is talking, signal disinterest, and will eventually put off the most determined of talkers. A far better way of dealing with an interviewee who is talking too much is to interrupt with another question in order to redirect the interviewee to a more relevant topic.

Much has been written on 'body language'. It is tempting to regard a wide range of behaviours as capable of interpretation. For instance, it is suggested that an interviewee who scratches his nose while speaking is not telling the truth. It may be that the interviewee's nose itches. There are some behaviours, however, that should be noted. Nervous interviewees frequently jerk their foot up and down at speed, and appear stiff and may present as excessively formal. If the interviewee looks away from you, losing eye contact as they deal with a difficult question, it may be that they are very unsure of what they are saying, or even telling an untruth. It is too easy, however, to assume that such behaviours are capable of interpretation by non-experts with any real degree of certainty. People from different cultures may exhibit behaviours which would send quite different messages to others from the same culture. For instance, the avoidance of eye contact can induce suspicion in one culture, while it may be a sign of respect in another. For those who wish to make a study of body language, there is a range of interesting books obtainable in most management or social psychology libraries.

Note taking

Brief notes may be made of important facts, but it is important to ensure that note taking does not become distracting. In selection interviews your notes form a record of information used in the selection decision, so interviewers should check that they have all the information needed to make an assessment. In history taking it goes without saying that as complete a record as possible should be taken, while at the same time paying continued attention to the patient. Showing them that you are listening may still be possible by making suitable noises of agreement or inquiry while you are jotting down your notes.

Key skills learning points

▶ The most generally effective interviewing technique starts with an open question, and is followed by a series of probing questions which develop the response. This saves you from trying to find the ideally worded question, which probably does not exist.

▶ Use a conversational, rather than formal, style to get the most from interviewees.

▶ Listening is the most critical of skills required by interviewers. Capturing and interpreting incoming information, and formulating probing questions, requires a high level of skill and concentration. The interviewee should also be aware of your interest at all times.

▶ Interpreting non-verbal cues can be a risky process unless you are fully trained in their analysis.

►3
Equal opportunities

Many employers adopt policies which encourage employees to give fair and equal opportunities to all candidates for job opportunities, regardless of their race, sex, disability, sexual orientation, religion, politics or age.

English law provides a basis for some members of society to claim redress for unfair treatment in the employment process in respect of certain of these conditions. Individuals within such groups may make a claim against an employer for compensation if they are treated less favourably than other applicants when being considered for first appointment, promotion or training opportunities.

It generally rests with the employer to prove that equal opportunity was ensured for all applicants, and even would-be applicants. It should always be the case that selection decisions are based on a rational, evidenced-based decision-making process, particularly as the employer might be called upon to prove the justice of the decision in an industrial tribunal. It is for this reason that your employer asks you to record reasons for your decisions at each stage of the selection process. Some doctors, such as women, certain ethnic groups, overseas doctors and disabled doctors, often fail to get short-listed or gain posts for which they are qualified. One of the main causes of underrepresentation of these groups can be attributed to lack of equal opportunity practices in recruitment and selection procedures (Allen, 1988; Esmail and Everington, 1993, 1997; CRE, 1996; BMA, 1997, 1998: Esmail and Carnall, 1997.

Sex and race discrimination

The Sex Discrimination Act 1975 and Race Discrimination Act 1976 are the main sources of legislation. European Union Directives have also affected the law in recent years. Men or women may claim compensation for unfair discrimination if factors related to their sex are taken into account, except where a genuine occupational qualification exists. This rare exception might mean, for example, a woman being recruited to model women's clothes. In all other circumstances the employer should be able to demonstrate, if challenged, that all candidates were treated equally, regardless of sex, marital status, parental responsibility or pregnancy. Sexual harassment—'unwanted conduct of a sexual nature or other conduct based on sex affecting the dignity of women and men at work'—is also a consideration in law. This has led to successful actions against employers where, during the recruitment process, a member of a selection panel has so offended an applicant as to cause them to bring an action.

Race is defined as including colour, nationality or ethnic origin. The structure of the law is similar to that for sex discrimination. Direct discrimination on grounds of race or sex is unlawful. This occurs when would-be candidates are prevented, or discouraged, from applying for a post for which they might otherwise be eligible.

Indirect discrimination occurs where a condition is applied equally to all candidates, but its effect is to reduce the chances of one group more than another. An age requirement of, say, 25–30 years applied to all applicants would exclude more women than men because women are more likely to take a career break to have children during that age range. This would constitute indirect discrimination, and provide good grounds for an action against an employer unless it could prove that the age requirement was a 'genuine occupational qualification'. Similarly, a restriction on religious belief, for example by excluding Hindus from a short-list, would be indirect discrimination against persons on the basis of their nationality as Indians.

Disability discrimination

The Disability Discrimination Act 1995 created employment rights for disabled persons broadly similar to those defined above. A person has a disability if 'he has a physical or mental impairment which has a substantial and long-term adverse effect on his ability to carry out normal day-to-day activities'. Organisations with 15 or fewer employees are exempt.

Disability has been widely defined, and includes, for example, severe facial disfigurement and progressive illnesses such as AIDS or multiple sclerosis. Employers may not exclude disabled candidates from employment opportunities without justification. They should make reasonable adjustments to normal working arrangements in order to accommodate the disabled person's needs. In addition to modifying premises, this might also involve adjusting working hours, modifying equipment or arranging special training.

In general, our advice is to try your best to treat all candidates in the same way. If you are concerned that a course of action you wish to take may be unlawful, always seek advice from your personnel or medical staffing department before acting.

▶4
Appraisal

Appraisal in context

Before any detailed exploration of the appraisal process can begin, it is necessary to define precisely what we mean by appraisal—within healthcare it has come to mean different things to different groups. Most doctors think firstly of appraisal as being related to the training process. In this case, it is seen as developmental rather than judgmental. Secondly, appraisal has now been introduced for all doctors, largely as a result of the perceived need to revalidate doctors on a regular basis. Finally, managers in the National Health Service are accustomed to annual appraisal as a means of assessing performance and, in many cases, determining career advancement and pay awards. Assessment is sometimes confused with appraisal. Calman introduced annual assessment for the specialist registrar grade. Thus, there appear to be four major types of appraisal or assessment. These, and their relationship with one another, are shown in Figure 4.1.

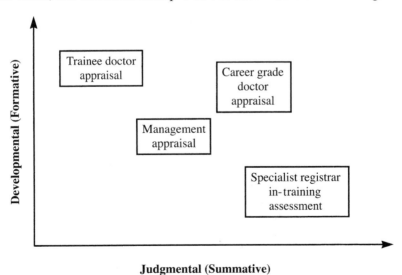

Figure 4.1 Relationship between appraisal and assessment systems used in the National Health Service.

Feedback on appraisal of performance, which is primarily aimed at helping the appraisee to learn and develop, is sometimes referred to as *formative* assessment. This may be contrasted with *summative* assessment, which seeks to measure ability in order to make an award, or to permit progress over a performance hurdle, such as in the annual assessment of specialist registrars.

The main aim of this chapter is to provide a basis for successful medical appraisal interviews, and in order to do this we must achieve a common understanding of the objectives of the two medical appraisal interview settings—for trainees and career grades. Each is separately outlined below, and contrasted with the other type of appraisal commonly in use throughout the Health Service—management appraisal.

Management appraisal

Formalised systems for the appraisal of managerial performance have been in common use in the UK since the 1970s. Their main objectives have been to identify management development needs, to create career and succession plans and to determine individual performance-related pay awards. This is achieved by reviewing the manager's performance against goals which are usually agreed on an annual basis. These goals are determined, as Figure 4.2 shows, by

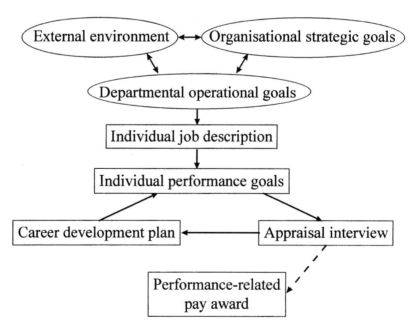

Figure 4.2 Management appraisal process.

reference to the organisation's goals, which are in turn a reflection of the environment within which it operates.

It may be seen from Figure 4.2 that one of the aims of managerial appraisal systems is to ensure that each individual manager's objectives are related to the overall organisational aims, and, in many cases, there is an obvious incentive to encourage the manager to achieve them.

At the heart of this type of appraisal scheme is the annual (sometimes twice yearly) appraisal interview. Such systems are attractive because they require managers to sit down and discuss their colleagues' performance in detail with them, including the problems they have encountered and their development needs. This meeting can take up to two hours, and is structured around the forms which review past performance, identify current issues, and set objectives for the coming year.

This approach contrasts markedly with the most common of medical appraisal interviews—the meeting between an educational supervisor and trainee.

Trainee doctor appraisal

Appraisal meetings should take place at the beginning, halfway through and at the end of the post. The first meeting is to arrange the training agreement, which sets out the learning objectives and confirms the support needed by the trainee during his/her time in the post. It is important that the trainee is properly prepared for this meeting, and guidelines for this are shown below (see 'Preparation—the trainee' below). The second meeting is primarily concerned with reviewing progress, designing new learning opportunities if they are required, and revising learning goals. The final meeting again reviews the trainee's experience, assists the trainee to reflect on experience gained, and helps to make sense of the complexities of the learning process. It will also address career-related issues.

We start from the assumption that enhanced education and development of the trainee provides the focus for appraisal at this level. It is, therefore, a *formative* process. Assessment, on the other hand, is *summative*—intended to determine whether or not a trainee is ready to proceed. There will be, of course, an element of assessment in any appraisal meeting, but trainee appraisal should focus on development, rather than judgement.

The Royal College of Obstetricians and Gynaecologists (RCOG, 1998) avoids using the word 'appraisal'—instead, it uses the term 'formative assessment' to describe its equivalent to appraisal. 'Summative assessment' is the final, or end-of-year, criteria-based assessment. Similar terminology is used by the Royal College of General Practitioners, and elsewhere in healthcare education.

There is no single set of guidelines to inform trainers of the 'correct' procedure to follow when appraising trainees. Information is available from the General Medical Council, the royal colleges, faculties, speciality bodies, deaneries, and trusts. Difficulties can sometimes arise in dealing with the information arising from appraisal—should it be kept confidential to the two parties to the appraisal, or become part of the evidence that is used to determine progress? There are schemes which encourage feedback from trainees on the quality and amount of training they receive. This can create difficulties for some doctors, who question the validity of such feedback. Other problems which arise relate to the ability of trainees to recognise their own weaknesses. This can give rise to conflict. These, and other problem areas, are addressed below. The following should assist you to decide which best practice you should adopt during appraisal.

Pre-registration house officers

The General Medical Council's *Good Medical Practice* (GMC, 1998a) provides the foundation for appraisal of pre-registration house officers (PRHOs). During their pre-registration year, they will normally be appraised on six occasions—three in the first six months, and a further three in the second. The very last of these might better be described as an assessment, since the decision to register is made on the basis of this final appraisal. It is not normal practice to record the outcome of the first three appraisals for the purpose of carrying forward evidence, so the final decision is often made without reference to performance during the first six months.

Each appraisal should consider four elements of the trainee's performance: clinical skills; communication skills; professional attitudes; and managerial skills.

Senior house officers

There are variations between royal college guidelines on the appraisal of senior house officers (SHOs), although most adopt a fairly common approach. Appraisal should be guided by the curricula of the royal colleges, and administered by the deaneries through clinical tutors and educational supervisors. SHOs should participate in audit by at least attending audit meetings, and may take part in projects. Appraisal should take place on three occasions during each post in a rotation—at the beginning (usually within two weeks), the middle and near the end. There is no consistent approach to the maintenance of written records of appraisal, nor is there a requirement that performance failings at earlier stages are communicated to subsequent educational supervisors in the rotation.

Specialist registrars

In addition to regular appraisal (three during each post, as with SHOs above), specialist registrars are assessed each year in accordance with their Record of In-training Assessment (RITA). The regulatory framework is set out in *A Guide to Specialist Registrar Training* (NHSE, 1998a), also known as the 'Orange Book'. Difficulty arises for educational supervisors when deciding the extent to which they should regard the appraisal as confidential, particularly when the final RITA assessment report is to be prepared.

General practice/vocational training scheme senior house officers

General practice/vocational training scheme senior house officers (GP/VTS SHOs) have three appraisals by an education supervisor in each six-month post, exactly as for career grade SHOs.

General practice registrars

There is an ongoing process of formative assessment by general practice trainers. Registrars should keep an educational log, which should contain a dynamic educational plan driven by the formative assessment process. This will obviously include regular appraisal by their trainer in addition to a formal appraisal after three months by the associate director. There are no national published guidelines on topics to be covered in appraisal, although the process is well documented by most deaneries. Additionally, the Royal College of General Practitioners, along with other appropriate royal colleges, has published booklets which detail the process and content of training in a range of subspecialities.

Appraisal and the learning process

Appraisal of trainees is, then, a formative process. Although some judgement is involved, it is normally intended that the trainee should be developed, rather than assessed. Appraisal is intended to be part of the educational process. Kolb *et al.* (1984) propose a model of learning which is useful when we consider the developmental role of appraisal (Figure 4.3).

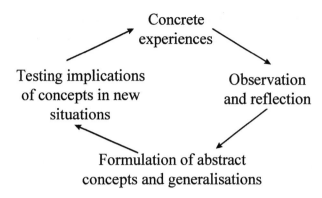

Figure 4.3   The learning cycle—a model of the learning process.

Concrete experience is gained through interaction with others—it suggests being involved in experiences and dealing with immediate human situations in a personal way. It emphasises *feeling* as opposed to *thinking*, and concern with present reality as opposed to theories and models.

Reflective observation is concerned with deliberation on the meaning of situations. It emphasises understanding as opposed to practical application and focuses on the *meaning* of situations and ideas and their implications.

Abstract conceptualisation focuses on logic, ideas and concepts. It emphasises thinking as opposed to feeling and is concerned with building general theories rather than intuitive understanding.

Active experimentation emphasises practical applications—what works, as opposed to what is absolute truth. There is always some risk associated with this stage in the learning process. It is about getting things accomplished.

Kolb *et al.* suggest that learning takes place when the learner follows the full cycle, for example, through concrete experience to testing new behaviours, after reflection and the development of concepts to explain the experience gained. Perhaps learning is initiated when the learner reads about a new theory or proposition. Only by testing out that proposition in real life, gaining new concrete experience and reflecting on it, can the proposition be modified in the light of experience, and learning take place.

A well-conducted appraisal meeting provides an opportunity for the trainee to gain important new *concrete experience*, through interaction with a senior colleague whose opinion is important to the trainee. The appraiser helps the trainee to *reflect* on experience, and also assists in the acquisition and development of *understanding of new concepts*. It remains for the trainee to go out and test out the learning in their own way, taking risks (under the supervision of a senior colleague) and acquiring new experience to reflect on later. For a more detailed explanation of how Kolb' *et al.*'s model helps you to understand learning in medicine, refer to Gatrell and White (1998).

Preparation for the appraisal meeting

Agenda

The following check-list should help you to prepare and conduct the appraisal. Choose from it the items you consider should make up the agenda for the meeting.

▶ *Education*—what, if any, examinations should be in preparation? What courses should be undertaken?

▶ *Academic/research*—is advice necessary on research projects, or decisions to be made regarding suitable research designs?

▶ *Clinical experience and skills*—what specified procedures does the curriculum indicate? What levels of understanding and competence are indicated? Is good manual dexterity and hand/eye coordination necessary? Is experience of clinical risk management a requirement?

▶ *Knowledge*—what is an appropriate level of clinical knowledge? Is knowledge or use of evidence-based practice a requirement?

▶ *Organisation and planning*—what level of ability to organise their own work and self-organisation are demanded of the trainee? Is participation in audit an element of the training at this stage?

▶ *Teaching skills*—should the trainee be gaining experience of teaching others and, if so, at what level?

▶ *Career*—should the trainee be helped to make career decisions at this stage? What help may be necessary? Would sharing your own experience be helpful to the trainee?

▶ *Personal skills*—the wide range of personal skills demanded in the work of a doctor are indicated below. Select those which you feel should be discussed with the trainee:
  • Interpersonal communication: rapport building, listening, empathising, persuading and negotiating skills.
  • Decisiveness: taking responsibility, exerting appropriate authority.
  • Team-working: cooperating with others, leading as required, seeking guidance.

- Flexibility and resilience: able to adapt to rapidly changing circumstances and cope with setbacks.
- Thoroughness: being well prepared, self-disciplined, punctual and committed to carry tasks through to completion.
- Drive and enthusiasm: committed to patients and colleagues, motivated to achieve, curious, displaying initiative.
- Self-managed learning: takes learning opportunities, reflecting on experience, seeking guidance and advice.
- Probity: honest, showing integrity and awareness of ethical dilemmas.

Preparation—the trainer

The aims of a trainee appraisal meeting are to identify relevant learning goals, to agree and commit to them, to reflect on and make sense of the trainee's past experience, and to agree and record actions based on the discussion. These might be for either the appraiser or trainee to implement.

The following guidelines are intended to enhance the quality of the appraisal for both parties.

▶ *Plan the meeting*—dates and times for all meetings to be held during the post should be determined well in advance.

▶ *Give the trainee advice*—the trainee should be helped to prepare for the meeting. After you have prepared an agenda (see above) you should show it to the trainee. The trainee preparation guidelines (see 'Preparation—the trainee' below) could be given to the trainee, and discussed a few days before the meeting.

▶ *Relevant materials*—such as the curriculum, timetable, job description, rotas, previous appraisal records and notes of feedback from third parties should be collected together and considered before the meeting.

▶ *Suitable venue*—a quiet room, guaranteed free from interruptions, should be used. Bleeps and mobile phones must always be switched off or passed to a colleague.

▶ *Sufficient time*—there is no 'correct' amount of time to set aside for an appraisal meeting, but it is unlikely that much will be achieved in under half-an-hour. Note that the appraisal must take place in protected time.

▶ *Third parties*—Discuss the trainee with other consultants, trainees, nurses, midwives, technicians, physiotherapists and others as necessary to gain a rounded picture of the trainee.

▶ *Feedback*—seek feedback from the trainee on his/her experience of the post, the teaching and your performance, as a trainer and appraiser.

Preparation—the trainee

Trainees should be aware that the success of the appraisal meeting depends on adequate preparation by both parties. The list under 'Agenda' above should help you to determine your most important topics. Trainees should ask themselves the following questions, and make notes to take to the meeting:

▶ *Work performance*:
  - Which areas of the work do you enjoy most?
  - Which tasks do you feel you perform the best?
  - Which areas do you find most challenging, and why?
  - How might you have improved your performance?

▶ *Skills/abilities*:
  - Reflect on your strengths and weaknesses.
  - Which skills do you have which you believe are well developed?
  - Identify those skills which need more development.

▶ *Learning objectives*: What learning objectives would you like to agree for the coming period of training?

▶ *Training*: Are there any specific training courses, or areas of need, which you would like to have addressed in the coming period.

▶ *Career*: What are the main career issues facing you at present. Are there still key decisions to be made? What help do you need with them?

Conducting an appraisal meeting

The pattern of the meeting, partly determined by the level and experience of the trainee, should be dictated by the trainee's needs. Effective appraisal means getting the trainee to identify their strengths and areas of need, and to propose ways of meeting the latter. Although guided by the appraiser, a successful meeting will feel to the trainee as if it has been led by his/her own priorities.

Agree the agenda

The agenda should have been determined in advance with the trainee's help, but it is worthwhile briefly re-establishing the aims, and key items for discussion. If a record of the previous appraisal is available, this should be used to inform the discussion at this stage.

Review past performance

Get the trainee talking as soon as possible. Use questions to open up issues, and probe to help the trainee to explore his/her own strengths and weaknesses in the light of his/her performance. Try to avoid being directive. Allow the trainee to describe his/her perspective on issues, and help the trainee to reflect by using open and probing questions. Focus on specific aspects of the work. Give positive feedback where possible, particularly as a balance to any comments on less successful aspects of the trainee's work. Giving feedback requires a high level of skill and sensitivity. It demands a careful blend of drawing out the trainee to describe his/her own strengths and, particularly, weaknesses, and being direct in explaining concerns which you have, and which the trainee does not appear to recognise.

Explore and agree current learning needs

The trainee should have identified key learning needs in advance, but these may need to be modified in the light of the previous discussion. It may also be affected by information you have obtained by third parties in preparation for the meeting. You should remember that the responsibility for the trainee's learning is a joint one. Avoid taking on a list of jobs which could be more suitably undertaken by the trainee. Make brief notes to ensure you can recall critical issues. Reflect on learning objectives agreed for the post.

Agree learning objectives for the next period

These should be 'SMART'. This means they should be:

- *Specific*—relate to specific tasks and activities, not general statements about improvement.

- *Measurable*—it should be possible to assess whether or not it has been achieved.

- *Attainable*—given the time available, it should be possible for the trainee to achieve the desired outcome.

- *Realistic*—within the trainee's capability.

- *Timed*—the next appraisal date, or earlier, should be agreed as the time for reviewing the achievement of the objective.

Review and record decisions

You may wish to make brief notes throughout the meeting in order to ensure that all the key points are reviewed at the end. It is vital that a record is kept of the outcomes of the meeting. This should be agreed at the end of the meeting, and a copy kept by both parties. It will prove useful at the next meeting, and may also form a useful document for the trainee to use as a record of progress in a logbook or portfolio.

Get feedback on your performance

It is not common for appraisers to welcome informal feedback from the trainee at the end of an appraisal meeting. Indeed, it could prove to be an uncomfortable experience. Nevertheless, if the relationship between the two has developed positively, it can be very helpful for the appraiser to get an immediate indication of the benefits gained by the trainee. Bolder trainees may even give constructive criticism of the training received and any weaknesses perceived by them in the scheme. While this may be difficult, it will undoubtedly help future trainees, and give the appraiser greater satisfaction in the long-term. Alternatives include written feedback forms, which are sometimes used by college tutors to route feedback to the royal college.

Dealing with difficult issues

Confidentiality

There are mixed messages from some sources regarding the confidential nature of the appraisal meeting. Typically, it is suggested that if trainees are to feel free to express concerns about their capability or commitment to a speciality, then the appraiser must indicate that he or she will maintain confidentiality. However, in some cases the appraiser is also the assessor, who is required to complete an assessment, in the case of specialist registrars, for the Record of In-Training Assessment (RITA). The final appraisal of pre-registration house officers is intended as the indicator of suitability for registration. In these and other cases, the appraiser/assessor is in a difficult situation if confidentiality is an issue. There may also be circumstances when the appraiser feels, in the interests of patient safety, that information about the trainee should be passed on to others.

Our advice is that appraisers should help trainees to recognise that confidentiality is limited by the above conditions, and that they will do all they can to support the trainee, while ensuring that the normal procedures are followed.

Conflict

Should serious conflict arise between an appraiser and trainee, it serves little purpose to attempt to resolve it, since the trainee will always be concerned that fair assessment is compromised. We suggest that a new appraiser should be found as quickly as possible.

Serious personal problems

Difficulties in appraisal may arise due to the serious nature of personal problems which afflict some trainees from time to time. It is important that the appraiser takes responsibility for ensuring the trainee receives suitable support in these circumstances. They should not, however, assume responsibility for taking on a counselling role, or becoming personally burdened with the trainee's situation. Occupational health officers or personnel departments can usually assist in such circumstances.

Lack of personal insight

Occasionally trainees seem to lack the ability to see their own weaknesses as others see them. This can be particularly true where there is a lack of interpersonal skill. It may also be that trainees are not able to see their lack of progress in developing clinical competence and judgement. It is important to distinguish between those who really are unaware of the negative impact they create, or the concerns of other staff at the inadequacy of their clinical practice, and those who refuse to admit to weakness in order to protect themselves from negative consequences. In the latter case, it is important to help the trainee to recognise the value of talking about their problems, since it may lead to better career decisions if they are struggling with the demands of the speciality in which they are working. Once again, the most helpful way to do this is to use open and probing questions focused on specific examples of their performance to get them to confront the problem. Those trainees who truly are unable to see their weakness, even after supportive questioning and gentle challenge, will only perhaps come to terms with their situation when they fail an assessment. It is crucial that the clinical tutor, and perhaps the postgraduate dean, is made aware of such problems at as early a stage in the training as possible.

Appraisal for revalidation

The introduction of revalidation has raised the importance of appraisal. Figure 4.1 shows the relationship between systems for the appraisal of doctors and trainees. It emphasises the extent to which consultant appraisal is a summative process, as well as being concerned with development. Although any system of appraisal provides a basis for determining education and development plans, at the heart of medical appraisal is the ultimate objective—to help to provide evidence which will determine whether or not the doctor is 'fit to practice'.

Revalidation

The General Medical Council currently defines three stages in the revalidation process:

▶ Profiling performance and appraisal.

▶ Five-yearly assessment.

▶ The General Medical Council decision regarding revalidation.

Performance profiling is about gathering the information. Every doctor has to maintain a revalidation folder. This folder is the basis of the annual appraisal and contains information about each of the elements identified below. It contains information on how well the doctor is practising, and evidence of continuing professional development.

A small group comprising registered doctors and lay people assesses the evidence collected in the revalidation folder, normally every five years. The group is required to satisfy itself that the doctor remains fit to practice, and makes a recommendation to the General Medical Council. The Council then makes its decision and communicates this to the doctor. It is assumed that any concerns regarding a doctor's fitness to practice will have been raised before the end of five years, if the appraisal is being undertaken properly. There should be no surprises at the outcome for any of the parties involved.

Effective clinical governance demands that employers oversee a systematic process which evaluates, supports and monitors the quality of clinical practice. Any revalidation process implemented by an employer must meet the requirements of the General Medical Council. Following registration with the General Medical Council, doctors are required to demonstrate that they are properly engaged in continuing professional development. They should audit performance outcomes, and take action to improve continuously the quality of service delivered to patients. The main instrument used to monitor doctors' performance is the appraisal process. Professional development portfolios are designed by the medical royal colleges, and maintained by all career grade doctors. These provide the evidence on which appraisal is based.

Although local appraisal systems may vary in detail, the main characteristics are similar. Professional development portfolios are kept up to date by individual doctors. They are scrutinised on a regular basis (usually annually) through an appraisal process.

Revalidation folder

The revalidation folder provides a basis for the appraisal. It includes the outcomes of annual appraisal as part of the evidence of continuing development and monitoring, which is at the heart of the revalidation process. It contains all the information which is submitted for assessment prior to revalidation.

The first section contains personal details about the doctor, and a description of what the doctor does. It should also describe any factors in their environment which help or hinder the provision of a good standard of care.

The major part of the folder addresses all aspects of their performance, and should be based on General Medical Council guidelines (GMC, 1998b):

▶ Good clinical care.

▶ Maintaining good practice.

▶ Relationship with patients.

▶ Working with colleagues.

▶ Teaching and training.

▶ Probity.

▶ Health.

Guidance on requirements for additional information will be based on advice from medical royal colleges and specialty associations.

The folder should contain information about the doctor's performance. This may be obtained from a range of sources, including:

▶ Patients—for example, through a patient survey.

▶ Immediate colleagues, such as partners or other professions—for example, through a peer-associate questionnaire.

▶ Managers, where appropriate.

▶ Colleagues who refer to, or accept referrals from, the doctor.

▶ The doctor, for example through a self-assessment questionnaire.

There should also be information on:

▶ Performance—through internal and external audit.

▶ Evidence of continuing professional development, normally in accordance with royal college guidelines.

▶ Critical incidents, where appropriate.

▶ Results of external assessments.

When completed for submission, the folder will contain information covering the past five years of practice, as a minimum.

Revalidation appraisal

The appraisal is conducted by a registered medical practitioner and includes, but need not be confined to, the revalidation folder. It should be regarded as a formative process. In addition to aspects of professional development, the appraisal process will also highlight areas of difficulty which may include practice condition, equipment and staffing levels. Arrangements for developmental or remedial action should also form part of the appraisal outcomes.

The GMC indicates that the appraisal should be confidential. This, it is assumed, encourages open discussion of weaknesses without them becoming major issues before remedial action can be undertaken.

Preparation

The process should involve, firstly, a review by the appraiser of the written evidence contained in the revalidation folder. This may involve brief discussions between the two parties to clarify points of detail. This will be followed by a meeting at which the appraiser is taken through the revalidation evidence and explores the issues which arise.

All the normal rules for ensuring that the meeting is successful should be followed. Both parties should set aside sufficient time. A suitable room, comfortable and free from interruption, is essential.

Conducting the meeting

Peer appraisal can be a difficult and sensitive process. It is important that both appraiser and appraisee are adequately prepared for the process through training. Core skills, which are largely those detailed elsewhere in this text, relate to the appraiser's ability to get the appraisee to open up about the successes and difficulties in their work. The re-validation folder will form the basis for the discussion, and the appraiser should be fully familiar with its contents. It is vital that discussion focuses on specific aspects of the work of the appraisee, and avoids generalities which fail to address critical issues.

Some typical problem situations may include doctors who:

▶ are nearing retirement, and are unwilling to take the revalidation process seriously;

▶ have been trying to cover all aspects of a speciality and failed to refer patients to more experienced colleagues for certain procedures;

▶ have avoided taking on board newer and more effective procedures because they are not prepared to devote time to self-development;

▶ are known for their rude attitude to patients and staff alike because they appear to believe that such arrogant behaviour is expected of them; and

▶ have provided revalidation evidence which fails to convince the appraiser that they are operating safely or effectively.

There is no easy way of dealing with these difficult cases. In general, it is first and foremost important to provide them with time and opportunity to recognise and talk about the specific problems which may have arisen from their approach. Patient questioning in the face of a refusal to admit there is a problem may eventually produce a result. It is not, however, the function of appraisal to *deal* with the problem, merely to *identify* it and, ideally, to *engage the appraisee* in planning ways of addressing it. Revalidation guidelines emphasise the importance of dealing with problems locally as they arise.

Meeting outcomes

The outcome, for revalidation purposes, is a statement placed in the revalidation folder which confirms that a satisfactory appraisal has taken place and identifies any development needs. Actions which are recommended should be set as objectives (see the guidelines above). Both the appraiser and the appraisee should sign the agreed statement. It will provide an action plan to the appraisee, and form part of the review material in next year's appraisal.

The five-yearly assessment

At the end of the five-year cycle it is the doctor's responsibility to submit the revalidation folder to the local revalidation group. If it finds the evidence acceptable it will issue a certificate. The revalidation group certificate is forwarded by the doctor to the General Medical Council in order to maintain registration.

The revalidation group comprises:

▶ A registered doctor with knowledge of the practice.

▶ Another doctor who does not know the practice (one of these must be of the same speciality).

▶ A lay person.

The revalidation group will take into account the seven general headings mentioned above (GMC, 1998a). If any of these areas are not relevant to a doctor's practice, the doctor is responsible for explaining this in the revalidation folder.

The revalidation group will also recognise the contribution of effective team working (GMC, 1998b) and will look for evidence of:

▶ Purpose and values.

▶ Performance.

▶ Consistency.

▶ Effectiveness and efficiency.

▶ Chain of responsibility.

▶ Openness.

▶ Overall acceptability.

Key skills learning points

▶ *Giving feedback*—negative feedback is made more acceptable if it is preceded by positive remarks about the appraisee. Even better, get them to tell you about the weaker areas of their performance.

▶ *Setting objectives*—all objectives should meet the criteria of being 'SMART'.

▶ *Dealing with conflict*—if conflict is not easily resolved, the trainee should be transferred to the responsibility of another trainer.

▶ *Managing the confidentiality issue*—confidentiality can be crucial in getting the appraisee to open up about their weaknesses, but it has to be clear that behaviour which contravenes GMC or other regulations will lead to disclosure to others.

▶ *Avoiding taking on trainees' problems*—these may be simply to do with training activities—the trainee should carry some responsibility for organising their own learning. Additionally, you should recognise that your role as an appraiser does not make you an expert counsellor. If serious problems are disclosed, refer them to someone who is equipped to help them.

▶5
Selection

The selection interview is one of a range of means by which information is collected about candidates. Other methods include references, logbooks, presentations, tests of various types and, of course, the application form or curriculum vitae. Interviews may be conducted by an individual or, as is the case in most medical appointments, a panel of interviewers. If such a panel is to be effective in getting to know much about each candidate, it follows that the members of the panel must be well prepared, skilled at questioning and fair minded. They must also be capable of working effectively as a team in this delicate process.

Practice in the management of the selection interview varies widely. Many organisations outside medicine avoid large panels because they are seen as cumbersome and often ineffective as a means of collecting data of sufficient quantity and quality to make such a critical decision. Panels of around three or four are usually regarded as the most effective. Tradition and the regulatory framework covering the appointment of consultants and specialist registrars combine to encourage large panels of up to ten members, or even more.

At the end of the interview, candidates' profiles are compared with a person specification in order to decide which, if any, is a good fit, and at least meets all the essential criteria defined in the person specification. Selection, by definition, involves a process of discrimination. It also provides the opportunity for selectors to emphasise candidate 'acceptability' (Townley, 1991), the so-called 'good chap syndrome', rather than considering suitability as it resides in person specification.

The NHS has attempted to standardise current procedures for consultants (NHS, 1996). Many health authorities and trusts also issue guidance. Implementation of equal opportunities policies requires an emphasis on good advertising practice and achieving a balance between limiting personal information required of candidates and monitoring of gender and ethnic origin of candidates and employees.

Equal opportunities legislation aims to ensure that discrimination does not occur on the basis of a range of characteristics which are irrelevant to the requirements of the job, which restrict selectors' choice and are unfair to applicants. The BMA (2000) states those key principles as:

▶ Establishing a systematic approach to recruitment and selection which is clear to both applicants and selectors.

▶ Having strict procedures which can be monitored.

▶ Specifying the requirements of the post, which must be non-subjective and related to the capabilities required to fulfil the duties of the post.

▶ Selecting individuals against those requirements.

▶ Training all those involved in recruitment procedures in equal opportunities, short-listing, selection and interview techniques.

Hospital medical staff are normally supported in the recruitment and selection process by medical staffing specialists. This support is often underused, or even marginalised (Lupton, 1998). This has sometimes led to the continued use of poor documentation, less well-structured procedures and, occasionally, selection procedures which would be incapable of defence in an action for unfair discrimination. A better working relationship between these two functions can lead to considerable improvement in the efficiency and effectiveness of medical selection. Figure 5.1 shows the many stages which make up the recruitment and selection process. Each of these contributes to the effectiveness of the whole. The interview represents a relatively small, although very significant, element.

Defining the job

The primary purpose of the job description is to inform potential candidates of the nature, demands and key elements of the job. This should help them to decide if they want to apply. If they are offered the job, the job description may be used to support the contract of employment. The exit discussion can provide insight into the challenges and attractions of the job.

Person specification

The person specification provides those responsible for short-listing with a template against which to consider candidates. It is crucial that the document contains enough detail to ensure that panel members can discriminate between applicants. Once again, the exit discussion with the outgoing post-holder can

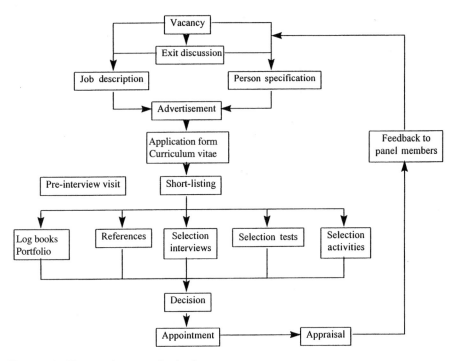

Figure 5.1 The recruitment and selection process.

be invaluable in providing information of the difficulties in the post for unsuitably qualified or experienced candidates. Our research indicated that incom-
plete or poorly drawn-up person specifications were frequently the cause of
major problems in the selection committee when the time came to arrive at
final decisions. In particular, the absence of adequate detail made it difficult to
engage in an informed debate about the strengths of candidates in relation to
the attributes demanded in the job. Details of those characteristics which were
most difficult to assess were often placed in the 'desirable' column, despite an
awareness that they were critical to the success of the appointment. These were
likely to include team working, leadership, self-management, professional
commitment and aspects of interpersonal communication. Recently, and particularly as a result of work undertaken at North Thames Deanery, a more
detailed, well-developed version of the person specification has been used in
the appointment of specialist registrars. An example based on the North
Thames Deanery version (North Thames Postgraduate Medical and Dental
Education Deanery, 1999) is shown in Figure 5.2.

All guidelines support the practice of sending a copy of the personnel specification to each potential applicant for information.

To applicants: you should complete your application form after carefully reading this person specification.

NORTH THAMES DEANERY
SPECIALIST REGISTRAR IN *SPECIALTY*
PERSON SPECIFICATION

	ESSENTIAL	WHEN EVALUATED	DESIRABLE	WHEN EVALUATED
QUALIFICATIONS	• GMC registration • MB BS (or equivalent), MRCP, MRCS/FRCS or FRCA, etc.	AF	• BSc (or other intercalated degree) • Other degrees/qualifications	AF
CLINICAL EXPERIENCE	• Relevant post-reg experience (SHO post in chosen field)	AF AF	• Experience in other related specialties • ATLS/APLS/ALS	AF AF
CLINICAL SKILLS	• Specified procedures— see Section F • Experience of clinical risk management • Competent to work without direct supervision where appropriate • Clear, logical thinking showing an analytical/ scientific approach • Good manual dexterity and hand/eye coordination	AF, Ref I/V I/V, Ref AF, I/V I/V, Ref	• Defined procedures—see Section F	AF
KNOWLEDGE	• Appropriate defined level of clinical knowledge • Shows knowledge of evidence-based practice • Shows awareness of own limitations	Ref I/V I/V, Ref	• Demonstrates breadth of experience and awareness in and outside specialty/ medicine • Demonstrates use of evidence-based practice	AF, I/V I/V
ORGANISATION AND PLANNING	• Ability to organise oneself and own work and prioritise clinical need • Evidence of participation in audit • Experience and ability to work in multi-professional teams	I/V, Ref AF AF, I/V, Ref	• Understanding of NHS, clinical governance and resource constraints • Active involvement in audit • Management/financial awareness especially of committee work • Information technology skills	I/V, AF AF I/V, AF AF
TEACHING SKILLS	• Evidence of teaching experience	AF	• Enthusiasm for teaching; exposure to different groups/teaching methods	AF, I/V
ACADEMIC/ RESEARCH			• Research experience, presentations, publications, prizes and honours	AF, I/V
CAREER PROGRESSION	• Appropriate progression of career to date	AF		
START DATE			• Available to start on *post start date*	AF, I/V
PERSONAL SKILLS	• COMMUNICATION SKILLS (clarity, intelligibility, ability to build rapport, listen, persuade, negotiate)	AF, I/V Ref		

	● DECISIVENESS/ ACCOUNTABILITY (ability to take responsibility, show leadership, make decisions, exert appropriate authority)	I/V, Ref		
	● INTERPERSONAL SKILLS (see patients as people, empathise, work cooperatively with others, open and non-defensive, sense of humour)	AF, I/V, Ref		
	● FLEXIBILITY (able to change and adapt, respond to rapidly changing circumstances)	I/V, Ref		
	● RESILIENCE (able to operate under pressure, cope with setbacks, self-aware)	I/V, Ref		
	● THOROUGHNESS (is well prepared, shows self-discipline/commitment, is punctual and meets deadlines)	I/V, Ref		
	● SHOWS INITIATIVE/ DRIVE/ENTHUSIASM (self-starter, motivated, shows curiosity, initiative)	AF, I/V, Ref		
	● PROBITY (displays honesty, integrity, aware of ethical dilemmas)	I/V, Ref		
	● LANGUAGE (ability to communicate effectively in written and spoken English)	AF, I/V, Ref		
PHYSICAL REQUIREMENTS	● Meets professional health requirements	● Pre-employment health screening		

AF = application form, I/V = interview, Ref = reference.

Figure 5.2 Example of a person specification.

Application process and pre-interview procedures

Application form or curriculum vitae?

Further developments are leading many organisations to require candidates to complete a structured application form in place of the traditional curriculum vitae (CV). This has many benefits, not the least being the ease with which those responsible for short-listing can discharge their responsibility. The application form can require candidates to respond to specific questions regarding their achievements in areas that are regarded critical to the post without waiting until the interview to discover such details. These might include level of clinical experience, experience of managing resources and level of actual involvement in audit. The extract shown in Figure 5.3 is again based on the North Thames Deanery Application form and shows two pages which are used in addition to the standard application form, and add considerably to the short-listing panel's ability to distinguish between candidates at this stage in the selection process.

Section G—Audit Management, IT

Please describe your experience of clinical audit. Indicate clearly your own level.

Please describe any experience of managing people and/or resources or of working in teams. You may give examples from both inside and outside medicine.

Briefly describe what you understand by the term 'clinical governance'.

Please indicate your level of familiarity with information technology.

Section H—Other Achievements

A range of personal skills have been identified as being particularly important in a successful medical specialist. For each of the skills indicated below, please give an example, preferably recent, from your own experience, to illustrate how you dealt with particular situations. You may draw from work or from other outside activities.

A. COMMUNICATION AND INTERPERSONAL SKILLS. (You need to be sensitive to the likely reactions of others to your actions. You must have the ability to work effectively with others and be aware of your own impact. You will need to be able to communicate clearly and present an argument persuasively.) In the space below, give an example of recent achievements that demonstrate that you possess these skills (up to 150 words approximately).

B. INITIATIVE. (You should be a self-starter. You must be able to determine priorities and to organise your time appropriately. You will need to take responsibility for producing results with the determination to see this through to a high standard.) In the space below give an example of recent achievements in this area (up to 150 words approximately).

Figure 5.3 Extract from an application form.

Short-listing

Consultants frequently complain of having to deal with very large numbers of candidates for training posts, and too little time to deal fairly with all candidates. If a standard application form is used, such as that advocated above, the numbers of applicants are reduced to those who are committed to trying to obtain the post. Alternatively, candidates may be encouraged, or required, to structure their CVs in a sequence to match the layout of the person specification.

Clearly, not all aspects of the person specification can be considered at the short-listing stage, but the more that are, the easier and fairer the process. Some advocate complex scoring systems for short-listing, others argue that criteria should be considered on the basis that candidates either possess them, or they do not. Any scoring system is seen as capable of being used to treat candidates unfairly. We have found a type of scoring which, we hope, accommodates both groups. Our suggested system for short-listing is shown in Figure 5.4. The person specification (above) indicates the items which may be assessed at this stage.

Weighting

Most panels prefer to weight items on the basis that some criteria are more important in making an overall assessment of the candidate in relation to others. Typical weighting scales run from 1 (lowest) to 5 (most important). The score (below) is then multiplied by the weighting to produce a more 'accurate' assessment. It should always be borne in mind that the system is far from

Post .... Assessor .... Date	Candidate Name -	A	B	C	D	E	F	G	H	I	J	K	L
Attribute (from person specification)	Weighting (optional)												
Basic qualifications													
Additional qualifications													
Clinical experience													
Knowledge													
Clinical skills													
Career progression													
Research experience													
Audit experience													
Management experience													
Communication													
Initiative													
IT experience													
Academic achievements													
Other													
Totals													

Figure 5.4 Example of a short-listing scoring profile.

foolproof, and the panel members, or a subcommittee, should normally meet to consider the scored outcome, and review those candidate profiles which fall just outside the short-listing range.

Scoring scale:

0 — Not up to standard now or in the foreseeable future.
1 — Not yet up to standard, but should be capable of reaching it through development activities before or on appointment.
2 — At the level required; appears to have all the credentials required for the post.

For those who argue that the *very good* should be distinguished from the merely *acceptable*, a further score may be used, although this brings the system into the range of some critics.

3 — Well above the level required for the job; would easily be able to accomplish the goals of the post.

Note that all decisions regarding short-listing will require evidenced written records.

Pre-interview visit

Such visits are regarded as solely for the benefit of the candidate, and should not form part of the selection process (NHSE, 1998a; BMA, 2000). Visits by applicants in advance of the interview have long been seen as an opportunity for their future colleagues to 'sound them out' for potential strengths and weaknesses. This has led to inconsistent treatment of candidates, who may have given out information in an unguarded moment which should not, in law, have been used to discriminate against them. If information gained informally is used, or even might have been used, to assist a selection decision, it would be difficult for an employer to demonstrate consistent and fair treatment of candidates.

References

The long-established use of unstructured references given by referees selected by the candidate is gradually giving way to employer-nominated referees, and structured reference forms. This approach is safer, and much more reliable. The example given in Figure 5.5 has been developed by the North Thames Deanery as a basis for the selection of specialist registrars.

This approach places responsibility on the referee to give clear advice to the selection panel on specific aspects of the candidate's suitability for the post. It also avoids the risk of error by omission. Note that references are shown to the

Name of candidate:

Applying for Training Programme for **Specialist Registrar** in:

Please complete your reference in the usual way, either using this proforma or attaching a letter.

Please also complete the structured part of this form as comprehensively as possible. The aim is to receive your professional view of the applicant with reference to specific attributes in the person specification.

Please give a summary view of your professional opinion as to the suitability of this candidate for this post. If you wish to enlarge on any of your comments above please do so.

Signed ....

Name ....

I. **Clinical Experience and Skills**

A. Do you have any concerns about this applicant's level of knowledge compared with other doctors at this level?

1. I have no concerns ☐
2. I have some concerns which relate to

....
....
....

B. Do you have any concerns about this applicant's overall clinical competence compared with other doctors at this level?

3. I have no concerns ☐
4. I have some concerns which relate to

....
....
....

C. Do you have any concerns about this applicant's awareness and insight into knowing when it is necessary to seek help/advice?

5. I have no concerns ☐
6. I have some concerns which relate to

....
....
....

D.   Do you have any concerns about this applicant's ability to organise him/herself and to prioritise clinical problems and his/her own work?

7. I have no concerns ☐
8. I have some concerns which relate to

. . . .
. . . .
. . . .

E.   Do you have any concerns about the manual dexterity of the applicant?

9. I have no concerns ☐
10. I have some concerns which relate to

. . . .
. . . .
. . . .

II.   Personal Skills

A.   Communication skills (clarity, intelligibility, ability to build rapport, listen, persuade, negotiate)
Do you have any concerns about the applicant's ability to demonstrate communication skills with colleagues and patients which promote teamwork and patient care?

1. I have no concerns ☐
2. I have some concerns which relate to

. . . .
. . . .
. . . .

B.   Decisiveness/accountability (ability to take responsibility, make decisions, assert appropriate authority)
Do you have any concerns about the applicant's ability to act decisively and take responsibility?

3. I have no concerns ☐
4. I have some concerns which relate to

. . . .
. . . .
. . . .

C.   Interpersonal skills (ability to see patients as people, empathise, work cooperatively with others)
Do you have any concerns about the applicant's ability to demonstrate interpersonal skills which promote good teamwork and which contribute to patient care?

5. I have no concerns ☐
6. I have some concerns which relate to

. . . .

. . . .

. . . .

D. Flexibility (ability to change and adapt, respond appropriately to rapidly changing circumstances)
    Do you have any concerns about the applicant's ability to demonstrate flexibility in day-to-day work?

7. I have no concerns ☐
8. I have some concerns which relate to

. . . .

. . . .

. . . .

E. Resilience (ability to operate under pressure, cope with setbacks, self-aware)
    Do you have any concerns about the applicant's ability to demonstrate resilience in day-to-day work?

9. I have no concerns ☐
10. I have some concerns which relate to

. . . .

. . . .

. . . .

F. Thoroughness (is well prepared, shows self-discipline and commitment)
    Do you have any concerns about the applicant's ability to demonstrate thoroughness in the approach to work?

11. I have no concerns ☐
12. I have some concerns which relate to

. . . .

. . . .

. . . .

G. Drive/enthusiasm (is a self-starter, motivated, shows curiosity)
    Do you have any concerns about the applicant's commitment, enthusiasm and drive for the specialty?

13. I have no concerns ☐
14. I have some concerns which relate to

. . . .

. . . .

. . . .

H. Probity (displays honesty, integrity, aware of ethical dilemmas)
    Do you have any concerns about the applicant's probity in the approach to patient care
    in dealing with colleagues?

    15. I have no concerns   ☐
    16. I have some concerns which relate to

    ....
    ....
    ....

    **Please note—a copy of this reference will be made available on request to the
    candidate**

    Signed .... Date ....

    Name .... Position ....

    Hospital/Trust ....

    Thank you for taking the time to complete this reference. Please return it to:

    Name and address of Medical Manager

Figure 5.5 North Thames Deanery structured reference form for applicants for the post of Specialist Registrar.

candidates on request. This should encourage referees to discuss it with the candidate. Most published guidelines suggest that this should be regarded as normal good practice.

Other selection activities

Tests

Selection tests fall broadly into three groups—those which measure:

▶ current abilities, knowledge and skills, such as driving or typing tests. Examinations fall into this group.

▶ aptitude or potential, such as numeracy or manual dexterity.

▶ personality.

Few tests are used in medical selection, although in many other fields of employment they are used extensively. Our advice is that, while tests can provide helpful insight into the strengths, potential or personality of the candidate, the results should be kept in perspective. They should only be considered in the context of all the other information obtained during the selection process. In most cases, discussing test results with the candidate can be extremely helpful for both.

Presentations

Short presentations on topics related to the appointment are being used more frequently as additional means of assessing candidates. While these can be informative, it is important to be clear about what the presentation is expected to reveal about the candidate, and how this relates to the post. If there is little or no demand for the post-holder to make presentations when appointed, then presentation skills should not be part of the assessment. It may, however, be helpful to ask candidates to present on a topic which relates to developments in the speciality, and to discriminate between candidates on the basis of their knowledge of the issues, or their clarity of thought. Criteria for assessment must be written down, and used consistently by all panel members.

Logbooks and portfolios

Most trainee doctors are aware that a logbook, or portfolio, can provide a useful basis for reflective learning. They can also be used as evidence in selection. As yet, few interview panels make much use of these as evidence of past achievement. If they are required of candidates, time should be set aside by suitably qualified panel members to review them, and relate the evidence therein to the person specification as a means of ensuring sufficient and relevant clinical experience.

Interview panels

Panel interviews for selection represent the norm in most large public sector organisations. Private sector selection procedures generally tend to use more one-to-one, or small panel, interviews, and combine these with other selection methods such as ability or psychometric tests. It is also more common for those with responsibility for selection to have received in-depth interviewing skills training. Where health authorities have provided training for staff involved in selection, medical staff are less likely than other groups to have received it (King Edward's Hospital Fund for London, 1990). Senior medical practitioners are less likely to be aware of the provisions of codes of practice and legal requirements. Where employing authorities have been found liable in discrimination cases, it has commonly been attributed to lack of training. Panel chairpersons and members should take responsibility for acquiring skills in interview techniques and an understanding of equal opportunities legislation (NHSME, 1993; BMA, 2000), as well as their own organisation's policies on equal opportunity. Our research (Gatrell and White, 1997a) showed the positive effect training can have on the performance of interview panel members.

Panel members should declare any personal interest in applicants which may be regarded as significant to the selection process. It is important that this is done at the beginning of the selection process and that new information is not introduced during the final discussion of the appointment.

Panel membership

There are no formal guidelines for the composition of interview panels for senior house officers and pre-registration house officers. Panel membership for the appointment of consultants, specialist registrars and general practice vocational training scheme is defined by NHS regulation.

Consultants

- Lay person, usually trust chairman or non-executive director.
- Chief executive of trust or representative.
- Medical director or consultant representative.
- Local consultant of same speciality.
- Royal college assessor (who has no right of veto).
- University representative (when the post has a substantial teaching or research commitment).

The above represents the minimum requirements for the panel membership. There is no statutory maximum. There is a recommendation that a majority of panel members are local, and medical.

Specialist registrars

Panel membership in England and Wales (NHSE, 1998a) should include:

- Lay chair.
- College faculty representative, preferably from outside the training area.
- The postgraduate dean or a representative.
- Representatives of consultants in training locations. Minimum two and maximum four.

▶ Local university representative.

▶ Programme director or chair of regional speciality training committee.

▶ Representative of senior management from a trust in rotation.

For specialist registrars in Scotland the panel comprises at least five members, including:

▶ Chair from a panel drawn up by postgraduate dean in consultation with trusts.

▶ Member from an appropriate section of National Panel of Specialists.

▶ Member of the regional postgraduate medical education committee (usually the postgraduate dean or representative).

▶ Senior medical representative of the services principally involved in the training programme

▶ A consultant appointed by the relevant university.

Senior house officers

Selection panels for SHOs follow no regulated set procedures. Recruitment of SHOs is often informal and undocumented, so that fairness and efficacy are difficult to assess. Sometimes a single consultant interviews and decides on the appointment. The short-term nature of some SHO contracts has tended to lessen concern. It should be noted, however, that these posts, so early in doctors' training, could have great influence on their later careers so the decision can be important. They are also subject to equal opportunity requirements and should normally be brought into the same local procedural arrangements as used for other appointments.

Pre-registration house officers

Most house officer posts are filled through medical school matching systems. Nearly all schools have schemes to match students to consultants. Posts and students remaining unallocated find places either by word of mouth or through the clearing-house scheme. Attention has been drawn earlier to the potential abuse of such systems. Equal opportunities arrangements in house officer appointments are improved if made by a properly constituted appointments panel, perhaps within a closed matching system.

Associate specialists

Until 1997, associate specialist appointments were usually personal appointments. They were not advertised, but were made on an individual basis. They were usually made to doctors already working in a trust and who met the criteria for permanent appointment. Appointments were established for those doctors who were unable to complete higher professional training, or who were unable to accept the full responsibility of a consultant appointment. Since 1997, however, posts in England may be advertised and associate specialists recruited directly by competition.

The recommended appointment committee should comprise, as a minimum, the following:

▶ A senior manager of the trust.

▶ A consultant (or associate specialist) from the trust, preferably in the same speciality.

▶ A further external senior hospital doctor nominated by the appropriate medical royal college or faculty.

For posts which have been advertised, there should be a further college representative. The trust may appoint extra members to the committee as necessary. Trusts, therefore, need to consider seriously the need for the post and whether or not a consultant appointment would be more appropriate. Appointment procedures are specified nationally, whether the post is advertised or not. A job description of the associate specialist post should be drawn up with advice from a representative of the relevant royal college or faculty.

Staff grades

The staff grade is a non-training career grade intended to provide a secure and satisfactory career in hospital medicine for doctors who do not wish or are unable to train for consultant status (NHSE, 1998a). Appointments following the probationary year may be held until retirement.

The advisory appointments committee for staff grades must comprise at least:

▶ A lay chair.

▶ A professional member from outside the district appointed on the advice of the appropriate college or faculty.

▶ A professional member employed in the district in the relevant speciality.

In certain circumstances employers may offer fixed-term appointments. These are for up to a period of five years, renewable each year. Job descriptions and contracts should be issued to applicants.

Senior clinical medical officers/clinical medical officers

These work in community health services and are roughly equivalent to associate specialist and staff grades. No appointment procedures are laid down, but the BMA advises recruiters to follow staff grade appointment procedures.

Locum doctors

All locum appointments either direct NHS or through locum agencies have to comply with NHSE Code (1997):

▶ Locum doctors appointments should be made with the same care as substantive appointments.

▶ Locum applicants who are in substantive posts elsewhere, or have held them within the last two years, should supply a reference from their employer.

▶ Trusts should introduce a structured assessment for references.

▶ Before first appointment, or when first registering with a locum agency, the doctor should undergo a formal health assessment by an occupational health department.

▶ Locums should be required to provide a statement of criminal convictions.

General practice partners

The panel normally consists of other partner(s) and a practice manager.

Single-handed general practices

In single-handed general practices the Family Health Services Authority (FHSA) or Health Board decides whether to short-list and interview candidates themselves or whether to appoint a selection committee to act on their behalf (NHSE, 1998b; DHSS, 1990), which usually involves a representative of the local medical committee (LMC).

Conducting the interview

The interview is a conversation with a specific purpose. This is to glean sufficient information about the candidate to enable the interviewers to decide, after combining this with other information obtained from elsewhere, to match the person to the job. It is guided towards its object by the interviewers. It falls somewhere between a formal meeting and a conversation. Practice in the management of the selection interview varies widely, although the structure of most medical appointment procedures is fairly formal (see above).

Selection interviews are most suited to determining that the candidate possesses an acceptable level of interpersonal skills and is committed to the appointment. The extent and quality of experience, evidence of capability, and gaps and irregularities in the application can also be checked.

Preparation

The best selection panels operate as a team. Members work together well, and have a good understanding of the roles and contributions expected of each. In order to achieve this, selection interviewers should plan carefully the structure and content of the interview. We recommend an hour of planning time, particularly for the larger panels (six to ten members) used in medical selection. Failure to plan properly can lead to the first candidate getting considerably less attention from panel members, as they shuffle papers in their attempts to catch up with preparation (Gatrell and White, 1997a–d). Preparing questions in advance will ensure that all the necessary issues are covered in the interview to enable the panel to assess individuals against the selection criteria in a consistent manner and make informed selection decisions.

It is good practice to set aside time before the interview, during which the chair will normally ask members to indicate priorities and concerns regarding the candidates. Discussion of the process is also important. If the sense of a 'conversation with a purpose' is to be maintained throughout the interview, then the flow of information must be managed with care. All members need to understand the chair's approach and agree their own contribution.

The panel should also agree on how members will be introduced to the candidate (they usually forget names and titles as soon as they hear them, if there are too many). Decisions on levels of detail, whether or not to shake hands, and who will collect and bring in the candidate, can have a significant impact on the time it takes to put the candidate at ease. Our experience suggests that candidates value being collected and introduced by one of the medically qualified members of the panel, rather than a junior administration staff member.

Candidates are often unskilled in presenting themselves, and doctors untrained at interviewing for selection. Some research has shown that inexperienced interviewers make up their minds very early, even within a few minutes of the start of the interview (Eggert, 1992). This leads to an interview in which questions are framed which serve only to confirm the interviewers' prejudices. It is important for the chair to discourage this approach by allowing time to discuss such issues before starting the first interview.

Timing

Perhaps the most common criticism made of interviewers is that they fail to manage the timing of interviews. Running late has a number of undesirable side effects. Unfortunately, this is such a common occurrence that it is taken for granted by panels and interviewees alike. The problem usually stems from an unwillingness to accept the fact that interviewing is a complex process, and takes a lot of time if it is to be done well.

Making an employment decision, which has critical influence on the lives and careers of the candidates as well as patients and colleagues in the hospital or practice, should be a slow and deliberate process. Sufficient time is needed, seldom less than an hour for each candidate for senior appointments.

Time should be allowed for reflection, discussion and writing up of notes between interviews, coupled with adequate time for discussion at the end of the interviews. Failure to do this leads to long delays for candidates who are scheduled for later in the day. This causes stress and prevents them from performing as well as they might. It also puts pressure on the panel and can lead to hurried, ill-considered decisions.

Room arrangements

Other issues for the panel to consider before the start include arrangements for the comfort of the interviewers and interviewee. Physical barriers may exist if the room is too small, causing candidates and interviewers to feel uncomfortable and cramped, or too large so that both parties can feel daunted. It may be too hot or too cold so that either party may feel uncomfortable. Untidiness can be a distraction, and the layout of the furniture with a large desk or chairs for the interviewers and a small chair for the interviewee is a power game to avoid. A large table can form a barrier but is common enough in medical interviews to be generally acceptable. The layout of the seating arrangement has a significant impact on the flow of information. It can also be a factor in enabling the panel members to work effectively together. In general, when the panel size is greater than three, the table should be oval (Figure 5.6). This makes good eye contact possible between the chair and fellow panel members. It also helps the interviewee to feel he or she is a part of the conversation, rather than the subject of an interrogation.

Selection interview structure

Interviews normally follow a pattern which emphasises the flow of information *from* the candidate *to* the interviewers.

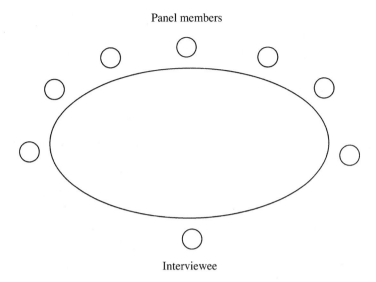

Figure 5.6   Room layout for panel interview.

There are four stages.

Opening the interview

The first stage lasts for about a minute only, and is concerned with making the candidate feel at ease and prepared for the process. This is often achieved by a brief, informal question and answer session between the chair and the candidate, or as a panel member collects the candidate from the waiting room, usually on an inconsequential topic such as the weather, the candidate's journey, or car-parking problems at the interview venue. Introductions are sometimes made at this stage, although candidates are unlikely to absorb information about names and titles. It is generally more efficient to leave it to individuals to introduce themselves when it is their turn to question the candidate. The point is made above regarding planned decisions about hand-shakes and so on.

Acquiring information about the candidate

The second stage commences within a minute or two of the start, and is the dominant part of the interview, taking up 90% or more of the total time available. This stage focuses on acquiring information about the candidate's life, educational and work experience, checking panel members' perceptions based on the application form or curriculum vitae, and exploring leads which arise in the course of the candidate's responses to questions. The focus is likely to be those attributes identified in the person specification which cannot easily be assessed by references, application form or other means, such as tests or presentations. This will include the candidate's interpersonal skills, team working, and other aspects relating to personality. The opportunity should also be taken to check on any uncertainties which have arisen following review of the application form. The success of the interview depends heavily on the skills of the panel members as questioners and, above all, as listeners.

Many writers on selection interviews argue that the only reliable indicator of a candidate's future performance and behaviour is what he or she has already done, and how he or she has carried out tasks and reacted to situations in the past. Getting the candidate to talk through the use of his or her skills and judgement in previous events tells us much more than asking speculatively about possible future events. Questions should focus on getting the candidate to describe and explain the ways in which he or she has dealt with particular situations which are relevant to the post.

This approach usually requires the use of an open question followed by a chain of probing questions, each of which are prompted by leads in the candidate's responses. Relevant techniques are described in more detail in Chapter 1 under questioning techniques.

Informing the candidate

The third stage of the interview gives the candidate the opportunity to question the panel. This should take up relatively little time, especially if pre-interview procedures have given candidates adequate detail regarding the job and organisation. It is unhelpful to take up the panel's time in giving detailed answers to questions about terms and conditions of employment. These are best deferred by the chair until after the interview, when a one-to-one meeting with a relevant person can save time and deal properly with issues of importance to the individual. It may be helpful to advise candidates in advance that the panel will not be impressed by being asked numerous questions which could have been answered outside the interview. However, it is critical that candidates are allowed to question the selection procedure, and express any fears they may have about the fairness of the process.

Closing the interview

Individual panel members may have noted an important query after their turn to question has finished, and may need to come back to the candidate with a further query. It is good practice for the chair to 'sweep up' any outstanding issues by inviting panel members to ask additional questions at this stage. Finally, candidates should be thanked, informed of the next stage in the process, and, if necessary, helped to find their way from the interview room. It is important to avoid time wasting. The chairman should prevent candidates (or panel members) from prolonging the interview with inconsequential discussion.

Assessment and decision making

The most difficult challenge facing members of the panel is that of reserving judgement until after all of the candidates have been interviewed. Sufficient time must be set aside at the end of the interviews to consider each applicant fully. In deciding on the merits of each candidate, rating scales for a range of attributes are sometimes helpful. The attributes might include personality, appearance, presentation, qualifications, experience, research, management ability and so on depending on the nature and level of seniority of the post. These will have been considered at an earlier stage in the process and should be recorded in the person specification. Selection criteria must be objective, job related, non-discriminatory and applied consistently to candidates. The panel should concentrate on facts, past performance and current circumstances using all available data including references and any test results. A table similar to that used for short-listing is normally employed, but with more details in those areas such as interpersonal skills, judgement, flexibility, resilience and, possibly, professional commitment.

The chair should ensure that all members of the interview panel are allowed to express their views about the candidates in an attempt to reach a consensus. Established theory on group dynamics indicates the importance of asking each panel member to privately note their choice, or ranked order of preference before discussion takes place. These noted scores should then be aggregated and only then should the outcome be discussed to reach a joint decision.

The decision should always be formally recorded. Reasons for rejecting unsuccessful candidates, and for accepting the appointment of a second candidate if the preferred candidate fails to take up the appointment, should also be recorded. Records should be retained for at least one year as they may be required if a complaint is made to an industrial tribunal. The panel must be prepared to reject all candidates if none is found to match the agreed requirements of the post.

The proceedings of the committee are strictly confidential. All notes, references and other documents must be collected at the end. If this is not done, individual panel members are advised to retain their own notes, in case of later action by a disappointed candidate.

Appointment

An authorised person should inform the successful candidate of the panel's decision. This constitutes an offer, and an acceptance by the candidate at this stage can create a legally binding agreement, an employment contract, unless it is made clear that any offer is subject to ratification by the trust board for consultants, or the postgraduate dean in the case of trainee doctors.

Care should be taken to ensure that all necessary pre-contract procedures have been followed. Failure to do so could lead to financial loss in a law-suit. It is good practice to make offers of employment subject to an occupational health assessment. The purpose of a pre-employment assessment is to ensure that the individual is fit for the job (Lunn and Waldron, 1991); for example, to ensure satisfactory hepatitis B status and to advise on the capabilities and limitations of those with disabilities.

Feedback to unsuccessful candidates

Giving feedback to unsuccessful candidates is often regarded as an essential part of the interview process. This is not generally the case in private sector organisations, other than for internal candidates. An appropriate member of the interview panel should be made responsible for providing feedback. It may be considered helpful to determine who will be responsible for feedback to individual candidates during the pre-meeting. This enables the panel member to note helpful feedback points during the interview.

Those called upon to give feedback should bear in mind the probable psychological state of the candidates. Most will be upset at having failed to obtain the post. Information for feedback should be based on this knowledge. They are likely to be sensitive to strongly adverse criticism. It should always be given so that the person:

▶ understands;

▶ accept;, and

▶ can do something about the information given.

This is best achieved by:

▶ focusing on being constructive—start with something positive.

▶ it is most helpful to deal only with a few (one or two) areas for action.

▶ concentrating on the highs and lows during the interview by referring to specific behaviour.

▶ concentrating on things within the individual's control.

▶ not overloading the individual.

If a trainee's serious shortcomings come to light during the selection process, these should be dealt with through the postgraduate dean or perhaps a relevant clinical tutor. Avoid addressing such problems at the end of the interview session.

Evaluation

A post-appointment review, perhaps a few weeks or months into the appointment, is good practice, although this seldom happens. Problems and failures at interview may be due to poor interview technique, lack of appropriate experience, an unsuitably constituted panel, poor chairmanship, unreliable references, or many other possible causes. These should be considered, by those responsible for managing the process, in relation to the appointee's performance. Feedback on, for example, the candidate's first appraisal should be routed to all those on the appointment panel.

Interview behaviours to avoid

Stereotyping

Untrained interviewers may sometimes ask questions that reflect stereotyping around assumptions made about particular groups of people. These might include, for example, assumptions that women of a particular age may be intending to start a family or, if they have a family, that they may be unreliable in attendance. It is sometimes assumed that all women are unable to carry out physically demanding work.

This is unfairly discriminatory, and may result in a successful legal action against a potential employer. Other assumptions arise around working relationships—that a woman working with men, or a man working with women, will cause problems, or that a black person working with white colleagues may have problems getting on within the team.

'Halo and horns' effects

The halo effect can occur when an interviewer is impressed by the fact that a candidate's experience or interest matches that of the interviewer, such as studying at the same school, university or medical school, or playing a sport in common with the interviewer. The interviewer may consequently spend time seeking positive feedback from the candidate to support this initial impression and ignore any negative evidence.

The horns effect is the reverse and occurs when a candidate shows interests or experience in their curriculum vitae which is not of interest to, or contradicts the values of, the interviewer. In this case, the interviewer subconsciously seeks negative evidence to support the prejudice.

Key skills learning points

▶ *Person specification*—this is the key document on which the success of the whole process is based. It needs careful preparation.

▶ *Pre-interview visits*—these are intended to assist the candidate. They should not form part of the selection process.

▶ *References*—the only helpful references are structured to ensure that the information obtained is relevant and complete.

▶ *Panel preparation*—adequate time (about one hour) should be set aside before the panel commences the first interview.

▶ *Decision making*—must be deferred until all information is obtained and interviews have been completed. Individuals should privately rank the candidates before they are aggregated and discussed to reach a final decision.

▶ *Situational questioning*—the real abilities and potential of candidates will only be reliably revealed by the use of open questions which focus on what they have already done. Probing questions should then be used to explore in more detail the candidates' strengths and weaknesses.

► References

Allen I (1988) *Doctors and their Careers*. London: Policy Studies Institute.

BMA (1997) *Meeting the Needs of Doctors with Disabilities*. London: British Medical Association.

BMA (1998) *The Future of our Doctors*. London: British Medical Association.

BMA (2000) *Recruitment and Selection of Doctors. Guidelines for Good Practice*. London: British Medical Association.

CRE (1996) *Appointing NHS Consultants and Senior Registrars*. London: Commission for Racial Equality.

DHSS (1990) *GP Practice Vacancies; Revised Selection Procedures, HN(90)26*. London: HMSO.

Eggert M (1992) *The Perfect Interview. All You Need to Get it Right First Time*. London: Century.

Esmail A and Everington S (1993) Racial discrimination against doctors from ethnic minorities. *British Medical Journal* 306: 691–2.

Esmail A and Carnall D (1997) Tackling racism in the NHS. *British Medical Journal* 314: 618–19.

Esmail A and Everington S (1997) Asian doctors are still being discriminated against. *British Medical Journal* 314: 1619.

Gatrell J and White A (1997a) *Appointing SpRs—Getting it Right First Time. Clinician in Management*, Vol 6, No 1. Cheadle: British Association of Medical Management.

Gatrell J and White A (1997b) Do you select doctors on science or gut feeling? *Medical Interface. The Journal of Disease Management* January: 24–6.

Gatrell J and White A (1997c) Selecting doctors—making the most of the panel interview. *Medical Interface. The Journal of Disease Management* February: 24–7.

Gatrell J and White A (1997d) Selection interview skills: so little time to listen. *Anaesthesia Points West. Journal of The Society of Anaesthetists of South West Region* Spring: 31–3.

Gatrell J and White T (1998) *The Specialist Registrar Handbook*. Abingdon: Radcliffe Medical Press.

GMC (1998a) *Good Medical Practice*. London: General Medical Council.

GMC (1998b) *Maintaining Good Medical Practice*. London: General Medical Council.

GMC (2000) *Revalidating Doctors—Ensuring Standards, Securing the Future*. London: General Medical Council.

King Edward's Hospital Fund for London (1990) *Equal Opportunities Task Force. Racial Equality: Hospital Doctors Selection Procedures*. London: King Edward's Hospital Fund.

Kolb DA, Rubin IM and MacIntyre JM (1984) *Organizational Psychology—An Experiential Approach to Organisational Behaviour*, 4th edn. Englewood Cliffs: Prentice-Hall.

Lunn JA and Waldron HA (1991) *Concerning the Carers*. London: Occupational Health for Health Care Workers.

Lupton B (1998) Pouring the coffee at interviews? Personnel's role in the selection of doctors. *Personnel Review* 29: 48–68.

North Thames Postgraduate Medical and Dental Education Deanery (1999) *Consultant 2000: A Competence Framework for Recruitment to the SpR Grade.* London: North Thames Postgraduate Medical and Dental Education Deanery.

NHS (1996) *HSG (96) 24. The National Health Service (Appointment of Consultants) Regulations.* Attaches SI 1996 no 701 and Good Practice Guide. London: HMSO.

NHSE (1988) *The New Hospital Staff Grade. HC(88)58.* Leeds: NHS Executive.

NHSE (1997) *Code of Practice in Appointment and Employment of HCHS Locum Doctors.* Leeds: NHS Executive.

NHSE (1998a) *A Guide to Specialist Registrar Training.* Leeds: NHS Executive.

NHSE (1998b) *GP Practice Vacancies: Revised Selection Procedures HSC 1998/227.* Leeds: Department of Health.

NHSME (1993) *Ethnic Minority Staff in the NHS: A Programme of Action.* London: HMSO.

RCOG (1998) *Professional Development File.* London: Royal College of Obstetricians and Gynaecologists.

Townley B (1991) Selection and appraisal: reconstituting 'social relations'. In: Storey J (Ed) *New Perspectives on Human Resource Management.* London: Routledge, pp 92–108.

▶ Index